The Needle Of Death

A story of death sold as life

By

Allen Wildisrael Makokha

Chapter One:: The Innocent Beginning

In the heart of Busakala, a place where the sun walks in tandem with its people, casting long shadows that whisper ancient tales, Linda, a bright-eyed teenager, found herself standing at the crossroads of tradition and the unforeseen. In Busakala, where footsteps resonate like a talking drum, the rhythms of life are steeped in a cultural symphony that dances between the past and the present.

As Linda prepared for routine vaccinations, the air in Busakala carried the weight of ancestral stories, where the sun bore witness to generations thriving in the arts of war and the alchemy of traditional medicine. Here, the people of Busakala had woven a tapestry of resilience, drawing strength from the very land beneath their feet.

The food they ate and the water they drank were more than sustenance; they were elixirs, believed to hold the power of healing. In this rich cultural tapestry, every bite and sip became a ceremony, a communion with the natural world that surrounded them.

It is within this vibrant yet enigmatic backdrop that Linda's innocence met the unfolding tragedy. The ritual of vaccinations, seemingly routine, now stood at the intersection of modern science and ancient wisdom. The collective trust of Busakala's people in the healing powers of their land would soon be tested, as the shadows of medical apartheid cast their veil over the unsuspecting town.

As Linda took those steps towards the clinic, the talking drum of Busakala beat a rhythm that echoed through time, signaling the beginning of a tale where tradition, science, and destiny would converge in ways no one could

In the heart of Busakala, where the sun painted the landscape in hues of gold, Linda, a bright-eyed teenager, was not merely a participant in the intricate dance of daily life but a cornerstone of her family's resilience. Born into humble economic circumstances, Linda's laughter echoed through the narrow pathways of the town, weaving a tapestry of joy amidst the baobab trees.

Linda's family, known for their modest means, found strength in their daughter's resourcefulness. She wasn't just a recipient of the town's traditions but a bearer of its economic hopes. With a deft hand in cultivating the rich soil and a keen eye for the marketplace, Linda played an integral role in supplementing the family income. The fruits of her labor, both literal and figurative, were intertwined with the vibrancy of Busakala's communal spirit.

The clinic, where Linda now stood on the threshold of medical advancements, was more than a venue for vaccinations; it was a meeting point between her aspirations and the economic heartbeat of her family. As the nurse's reassuring needle approached, Linda's resilience mirrored the strength of Busakala itself—a town where every member played a crucial role in the collective narrative.

Her economic contributions extended beyond her immediate family, reaching into the fabric of Busakala's society. Linda's expertise in traditional farming methods and her knack for resourcefulness made her not just useful to her family but a beacon of hope for others seeking sustenance and economic stability.

As we delve deeper into the intersection of tradition, science, and the unfolding tragedy, Linda's economic background emerges as a thread that ties her fate to the very economic pulse of Busakala. Little did she know that the innocent vaccinations would not only test her physical resilience but also challenge the economic foundation she represented in the intricate tapestry of her town.

The Reassuring Needle

Inside the pristine walls of Busakala's clinic, a sacred space where the scent of traditional herbs mingled with antiseptic, Linda found herself seated, her anticipation palpable. The nurse, a guardian of health in this small town, approached with a reassuring needle – a slender messenger carrying the promise of protection against the looming specters of polio and measles.

The gentle touch of the nurse mirrored the tenderness Busakala bestowed upon its own. "Fear not, Linda," the nurse's assuring words resonated like a comforting melody. "This is the shield that wards off unseen adversaries, ensuring a path to health and prosperity."

In another corner of the clinic, Dr. Masinde, the revered figure among Busakala's medical professionals, addressed the gathering with words that echoed through the chamber. "Dear people of Busakala," he began, his voice carrying the weight of experience and reassurance. "In this convergence of tradition and modernity, we stand united against the shadows that may linger. These vaccines are not just safeguards; they are gateways to a future where health and heritage coexist."

The words of Dr. Masinde were a balm to the collective anxiety that hung in the air. His encouragement resonated with the people, instilling a sense of confidence in the path they were undertaking. The clinic, adorned with murals depicting the harmonious dance between traditional healing and modern medicine, became a stage where the symphony of hope played out.

Little did Linda and her fellow townspeople know that these assuring words, meant to calm the currents of uncertainty, would become threads in a narrative that unfolded beyond the clinic's walls. The reassuring needle, coupled with the wisdom of Dr. Masinde, now stood as symbols not only of protection but also of unwitting participation in a story that would test the very foundations of Busakala's health and resilience.

III. The Unraveling

A. Linda's Health Deterioration and Mysterious Symptoms

As the days pressed on, Linda's vitality dwindled, leaving her grappling with an inexplicable descent into illness. The once-lively spirit of Busakala's narrow pathways was now a mere whisper in Linda's weakened frame. Fatigue clung to her like a heavy cloak, and fevers cast shadows over what were once sunlit afternoons.

Yet, it wasn't just the visible symptoms that tormented Linda. A persistent cough echoed through the night, a disconcerting soundtrack to her restless sleep. Limbs that once danced with agility now moved with hesitant steps, as though burdened by an invisible weight. Busakala, unwittingly drawn into the orbit of an unforeseen adversary, felt the ripples of unease as Linda's health continued to unravel.

B. Medical Professionals' Confusion and Attempts to Diagnose

Linda's family, growing increasingly alarmed, sought refuge within the familiar walls of Busakala's clinic. Dr. Masinde, a stalwart figure in the town's medical landscape, found himself facing an intricate puzzle of symptoms that defied easy explanation. Medical professionals, once confident in their ability to heal, were now confronted by the perplexity of Linda's case.

Tests were conducted, each result scrutinized with furrowed brows, yet a definitive diagnosis remained elusive. The clinic, once a sanctuary of healing, now hummed with the discordant notes of uncertainty.

Whispers of Linda's medical anomalies circulated, casting a somber tone over the very place meant to bring solace.

As Dr. Masinde delved deeper into Linda's case, the unsettling truth emerged – HIV and AIDS, words laden with profound implications. The once-reassuring needle, a symbol of protection, had inadvertently woven Linda into the intricate fabric of a medical enigma. The clinic's atmosphere shifted from one of reassurance to shared disbelief, as the medical professionals faced the harsh reality that the very act intended to safeguard had ushered in a heartbreaking transformation.

The revelation of Linda's condition sent shockwaves beyond the walls of Busakala's clinic. An investigation unveiled a staggering revelation: 700 other patients, recipients of the same vaccine, shared a similar trajectory. Each one, like Linda, found themselves ensnared in the unintended consequences of medical progress. The once-promising shield against polio and measles had become a gateway to a health crisis that extended far beyond the individual tragedies of Busakala. The town, once a beacon of resilience, now grappled not only with Linda's plight but also with the haunting realization that they stood at the epicenter of a wider health catastrophe, a storm they had unwittingly unleashed upon themselves.

IV. The Shocking Revelation

A. Linda's Diagnosis with HIV and AIDS

The once-bustling corridors of Busakala's clinic fell into an eerie hush as Dr. Masinde, with a heavy heart, uttered the words that would forever alter Linda's destiny. HIV and AIDS, whispered in a tone that echoed through the chambers, struck like a thunderbolt. Linda's diagnosis, once shrouded in mystery, now bore a name that carried the weight of a global health crisis.

In the quiet room, Linda grappled with the staggering reality of her condition. The vibrant threads of her life were now woven into the somber tapestry of a pandemic, a revelation that rippled through Busakala like a seismic wave. The once-reassuring needle, intended to protect, had unwittingly become the harbinger of a devastating illness, leaving Linda and her town in the grip of an unfathomable sorrow.

B. Uncover the Deliberate Actions and Manipulations by Pharmaceutical Companies During Medical Apartheid

As Busakala grappled with the shockwaves of Linda's diagnosis, an investigation uncovered a chilling truth – the deliberate actions and manipulations orchestrated by pharmaceutical companies during the era of medical apartheid. Behind the veil of progress and innovation lay a shadowy landscape where corporate interests eclipsed ethical boundaries.

The vaccines administered to Linda and 700 others were not the result of benevolent scientific endeavors but pawns in a calculated game. Pharmaceutical companies, driven by greed and a ruthless pursuit of profit, had exploited vulnerable communities during medical apartheid. The once-trusted guardians of health were exposed as architects of a silent epidemic, turning routine inoculations into conduits of unimaginable suffering.

The revelation laid bare a disturbing reality – the very entities entrusted with safeguarding health had betrayed the trust of communities like Busakala. The deliberate actions of these pharmaceutical giants, manipulating medical advancements for financial gain, became a dark stain on the canvas of progress. As Busakala grappled not only with Linda's diagnosis but also with the malevolent forces that had shaped their fate, a collective resolve emerged to seek justice and hold those responsible for the silent epidemic accountable.

In the unfolding chapters, Busakala faced a dual battle –against the ravages of HIV and AIDS and the shadows of manipulation that lingered over their town. Linda's story, now a symbol of resilience and defiance, became a rallying cry for justice and a testament to the town's unwavering spirit in the face of adversity.

V. Linda's Struggle

A. Linda's Emotional and Physical Battle Against the Devastating Effects

As the diagnosis of HIV and AIDS settled into the fabric of Linda's life, she embarked on a poignant journey, a battle that extended far beyond the physical realm. Emotionally resilient yet vulnerable, Linda faced the relentless onslaught of symptoms with unwavering courage. The once-lively girl, whose laughter echoed through the narrow pathways of Busakala, now confronted the specter of a relentless illness.

Linda's days became a dance with fatigue, her nights haunted by the persistent cough that echoed through the silence. The vibrant threads of her life were now woven into a tapestry of pain, yet amid the darkness, Linda clung to resilience. Each day was a testament to her strength, as she navigated the complex landscape of antiretroviral treatments, seeking solace in the hope for a brighter tomorrow.

B. Highlight Societal Stigma and Discrimination Faced by Linda

However, Linda's struggle extended beyond the confines of her own body; it became entwined with the societal stigma and discrimination that cast a long shadow over those living with HIV and AIDS. Busakala, once a tight-knit community, now grappled with prejudices that threatened to fracture its communal bonds.

Whispers and sidelong glances followed Linda, as if the weight of the town's judgment bore down upon her frail shoulders. The stigma, born from fear and misinformation, manifested in the isolation Linda faced from some quarters of Busakala. Doors that once opened freely now closed with a hesitant creak, and once-warm smiles turned into guarded glances.

Linda's emotional battle extended beyond her own resilience; it became a testament to the resilience of Busakala itself. The town, now faced with the harsh realities of societal discrimination, found itself at a crossroads. Would it succumb to the divisive forces fueled by fear, or would it rise above, embracing Linda as one of its own?

In this chapter of Linda's struggle, the emotional and societal dimensions intertwine, creating a narrative that goes beyond the individual to expose the collective strength or fragility of a community faced with a silent epidemic. As Linda fought not only against the devastating effects of the illness but also against the shadows of stigma, the town of Busakala grappled with defining its character in the face of adversity.

VI. Uncovering the Conspiracy

A. Investigative Journey to Expose the Calculated Moves by Pharmaceutical Companies

Fueled by a collective determination to unearth the truth, Busakala initiated an investigative journey, peeling back the layers of deception that shrouded the town in an epidemic born of calculated moves by pharmaceutical companies. Driven by an insatiable thirst for justice, a group of relentless individuals embarked on a quest to expose the sinister machinations that had left Linda and countless others in the grip of a devastating illness.

The investigative journey led them down a labyrinth of corporate intrigue, revealing a trail of deliberate actions and manipulations. Documents were scrutinized, whistleblowers sought, and the town's leaders collaborated with international agencies to shine a light on the shadowy practices that had exploited vulnerable communities during medical apartheid.

B. Unveiling the Broader Implications of Medical Apartheid and Unethical Practices

As the investigation unfolded, Busakala unraveled the broader implications of medical apartheid and the unethical practices that had woven a silent epidemic into the fabric of global health. The town, once a microcosm of suffering, now stood as a symbol of resilience against the systemic injustices perpetuated by pharmaceutical giants.

The shocking revelation came not only from within Busakala's confines but also from a confession that sent shockwaves beyond its borders. On live television, the French minister, a key figure in the global health landscape, admitted to the unthinkable – vaccines given to African children and women had been intentionally tainted to induce HIV and AIDS. The collective gasp that reverberated through Busakala encapsulated the magnitude of the betrayal.

Simultaneously, humanitarian organizations brought forth compelling evidence suggesting that the vaccines might indeed be the lead cause of the virus. The very entities entrusted with safeguarding health were implicated in a crime against humanity, challenging the foundations of trust in medical advancements and fueling a global outcry for accountability.

In this chapter of Busakala's story, the investigative journey unveils a web of deceit, exposing the calculated moves that had thrust the town into the heart of a medical crisis. The broader implications echo far beyond its narrow pathways, sparking a reckoning with the ethical boundaries of the pharmaceutical industry and laying bare the systemic flaws that had perpetuated a silent epidemic on a global scale.

VII. Seeking Justice

A. Linda's Quest for Accountability and Justice

In the face of the insidious conspiracy that had befallen Busakala, Linda's quest for accountability and justice evolved into a powerful force, transcending her personal struggle with HIV and AIDS. Driven by an unrelenting spirit, she became the voice of a town that refused to be silenced, embarking on a poignant journey to expose the truth behind the calculated moves of pharmaceutical companies.

Linda's advocacy stretched beyond the confines of Busakala, resonating with global communities affected by the same silent epidemic. Armed with resilience and a determination to ensure that her suffering and the suffering of countless others would not be forgotten, Linda navigated the intricate landscape of legal avenues, becoming a symbol of courage against corporate betrayal.

B. Legal Battles and Challenges in a System Intertwined with Corporate Influence

As Linda pressed forward in her pursuit of justice, she encountered legal battles that mirrored the complexities of a system intertwined with corporate influence. The legal arena became a battleground, where the very entities implicated in the conspiracy wielded considerable power. Obstructive legal maneuvers and attempts at discrediting witnesses became common tactics, revealing the formidable adversary that Busakala faced in its quest for accountability.

The legal challenges were exacerbated by a damning revelation – medical research had unequivocally marked the vaccine as unsafe for use by medical professionals. Despite clear warnings from dissenting scientists, corporations and governments, entangled in a web of corruption, allowed the vaccines to be used indiscriminately. The pursuit of profit and power had overridden the imperative to protect public health.

The ignored warnings became a pivotal element in Busakala's legal battles, exposing a dark underbelly of corruption that permeated the corridors of power. Linda's journey, entwined with the collective struggle of her town, laid bare the stark reality that justice faced not only legal intricacies but also the pervasive influence of corporate entities willing to sacrifice lives for financial gain.

In this chapter of seeking justice, Linda's courageous advocacy becomes a beacon of hope, shedding light on a systemic failure that went beyond the borders of Busakala. The legal battles, intertwined with the damning evidence of ignored warnings, symbolize a broader fight against corruption and corporate malfeasance, challenging the very foundations of a system that had allowed a silent epidemic to unfold.

In the twisted web of seeking justice, pharmaceutical companies and corporations, wielding immense power and influence, orchestrated a malevolent dance to silence the information that could have served as a beacon of truth for Linda and the 700 others entangled in the silent epidemic.

Behind closed doors, corporate entities, fueled by avarice and a desire to protect their bottom line, manipulated the course of justice. Legal maneuvers became a strategic tool to obfuscate evidence and bury dissenting voices. Lawyers, entangled in the web of corporate influence, utilized their expertise not to seek truth but to craft narratives that shielded the perpetrators from accountability.

Whistleblowers who dared to expose the conspiracy found themselves facing a barrage of threats and intimidation. The corporate machinery, well-oiled and relentless, spared no effort to discredit these courageous individuals, painting them as conspirators seeking personal gain rather than truth-seekers aiming to unveil a grave injustice.

Information that could have been a lifeline for Linda and the 700 others, revealing the deliberate actions that led to their suffering, was systematically suppressed. Studies and research that marked the vaccines as unsafe were buried under the weight of corporate interests. Scientists who raised their voices faced professional ruin, their credibility tarnished by a system that valued profit over public health.

The corridors of power, entwined with corporate influence, became echo chambers of complicity. Governments, lured by financial incentives and political alliances, turned a blind eye to the damning evidence that could have shifted the tide of justice in favor of the afflicted. The information that could have been a catalyst for accountability was muffled by the juggernaut of corporate interests.

In this chapter of Busakala's saga, the relentless pursuit of justice faced not only legal battles but a pervasive campaign to silence truth. The pharmaceutical companies, through their vast influence and financial clout, sought to bury the information that would have brought solace to Linda and the 700 others, leaving them trapped in a cycle of suffering and corporate betrayal. Linda's quest for justice, now entangled in a labyrinth of deceit, mirrored a broader struggle against a system that prioritized profits over the lives it had irreversibly affected.

VIII. The Ripple Effect

A. Explore the Impact on Others Who Fell Victim to Similar Schemes

The ripple effect of Busakala's silent epidemic extended far beyond its borders, casting a shadow over countless individuals who fell victim to similar schemes orchestrated by pharmaceutical companies. Families in distant communities, their lives intertwined with the promise of medical advancements, faced the devastating consequences of a betrayal echoing Busakala's tragedy.

In corners of the world unknown to Busakala, individuals who received tainted vaccines experienced health crises that mirrored Linda's plight. The silent epidemic, an unintended consequence of corporate greed and manipulation, became a global affliction, leaving communities grappling with illness, loss, and shattered trust in the very institutions meant to safeguard their well-being.

B. Raise Questions About the Ethics and Transparency Within the Pharmaceutical Industry

As Busakala's story reached the global stage, questions emerged about the ethics and transparency within the pharmaceutical industry. The saga exposed a dark underbelly where profit motives superseded ethical considerations, and transparency became a casualty in the pursuit of financial gain.

Corruption within pharmaceutical companies reached insidious depths, infiltrating not only research and development but also regulatory processes. The influence these corporations wielded over governments and justice systems became a disconcerting reality, raising fundamental questions about the integrity of the institutions responsible for protecting public health.

The labyrinth of corruption extended to cozy relationships between pharmaceutical lobbyists and policymakers. Campaign contributions and revolving-door dynamics blurred the lines between public service and corporate interests, allowing the industry to shape regulations in its favor. The very institutions designed to ensure the safety and efficacy of medical interventions became marionettes, dancing to the tunes played by pharmaceutical giants.

In courtrooms, legal battles faced by victims were often tilted in favor of the corporations, showcasing the extensive reach of their influence. The pharmaceutical industry's tentacles entwined with justice systems, manipulating proceedings and stifling dissent. Whistleblowers faced not only legal battles but also a relentless campaign of character assassination, discouraging others from coming forward and exposing the truth.

Governments, dependent on pharmaceutical companies for medical innovations and economic contributions, hesitated to hold them accountable. The cozy relationships between corporations and political leaders fostered an environment where the industry's interests superseded the public good. The very institutions entrusted with protecting citizens now stood compromised, entangled in a web of corruption that reached far beyond Busakala's tragedy.

In this chapter of the ripple effect, the story of Busakala transcends its narrow confines, becoming a damning indictment of an industry where ethical considerations and transparency have been sacrificed at the altar of profit. The pervasive corruption within pharmaceutical companies, influencing governments and justice systems, serves as a clarion call for a global reckoning with a system that has failed in its duty to prioritize the health and well-being of individuals over corporate gain.

IX. Conclusion

A. Linda's Legacy and the Lessons Learned from Her Ordeal

As Busakala's story reaches its conclusion, Linda's legacy emerges not as a tale of defeat but as a testament to resilience and the unyielding spirit of those who refuse to be silenced. Her journey, fraught with pain and betrayal, becomes a rallying cry for justice and a reminder that even in the face of insurmountable odds, individuals can spark movements that transcend their personal suffering.

Linda's legacy echoes through the narrow pathways of Busakala, inspiring a generation to question, challenge, and seek accountability. The town, scarred but not defeated, stands as a living testament to the strength that emerges from adversity. Linda's ordeal becomes a beacon, guiding others to navigate the intricate dance between progress and ethics, and to stand against the shadows of corporate malfeasance.

B. Encourage Readers to Critically Examine the Intersection of Science, Ethics, and Corporate Interests in Medical Advancements

Busakala's narrative serves as a cautionary tale, urging readers to critically examine the intricate intersection of science, ethics, and corporate interests in the realm of medical advancements. The story unveils the consequences of a system where the pursuit of profit often eclipses ethical considerations, leaving unsuspecting communities in the wake of a silent epidemic.

Readers are encouraged to question the narratives woven by pharmaceutical giants and to scrutinize the motivations that drive medical innovations. The lessons learned from Busakala underscore the imperative for transparency, ethical conduct, and a reevaluation of the power dynamics that often silence dissenting voices in the pursuit of progress.

As the final pages of Busakala's story turn, the hope is that Linda's legacy becomes a catalyst for change. A change in how society views the intersection of science and corporate interests, a change in how governments regulate and protect their citizens, and a change in how individuals advocate for their rights in the face of systemic injustices. In the aftermath of Linda's ordeal, the call to critically examine the ethical foundations of medical advancements becomes not just a narrative conclusion but an urgent plea for a world where progress is synonymous with the well-being of humanity, not the pockets of corporations.